Elemental

The Author

Paul Reed has lived in Muirhouse, Edinburgh all his life. In 1987, he began to experience various symptoms of mental illness and was diagnosed with schizophrenia in 2001. He drew on these experiences to write his acclaimed debut novel *The One*, also published by Mercat Press. He is now in great demand as a public speaker on mental health issues.

Paul Reed can be contacted c/o Mercat Press, 10 Coates Crescent, Edinburgh EH3 7AL, or by emailing *enquiries@mercatpress.com*.

Elemental

The Universal Art of Mental Health

PAUL REED

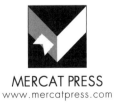

MERCAT PRESS
www.mercatpress.com

First published in 2006 by Mercat Press
Mercat Press, 10 Coates Crescent, Edinburgh EH3 7AL
www.mercatpress.com

ISBN 10: 1841831093
ISBN 13: 9781841831091

Set in Myriad Roman at Mercat Press
Printed and bound in Great Britain by
Bell & Bain Ltd., Glasgow

Dedicated to the Spirits of...

Sandy Cunningham, Ethel Ward, Mac from Muirhouse Library, Wee Gabby 'Skippy' Reed, and to my beautiful wee cat, Puddin the pudge, for showing me the meaning of unconditional love. Ah'll no' forget you, ma bonny lass. Dad loves that baby.

WISH YOU WERE HERE.

Thanks to...

Rita Rae, Simon Bradstreet at the Scottish Recovery Network, Wayne Turner, Arthur Howie, Flap and Laura, Lynn McKnight at STV, Clark Semple, Martha Thom, Maggie Reed, Geoff Thompson, Kieran and Aaron Logue, Keegs, Donna Anderson, Natty Beans Hill, El and Brian Hill, Gary Thompson, Carol Gillies, Ian Thompson, Bobby Summers and Gracey, James Wright and Colin McColl, Doory, Dougie and Juney, Everybody from Mexi's, Coco Adams, Maggi Morrison, Jeanette Stevenson, Mikey Haddow and the shopping centre party people, Jimmy Butler, Cha Lewis, Big Stan, all my pals in the mental health sector, Big Al and the Gunner mob, and to Joe who dances in the shadow of the Rainmaker. Love always to Esme Vincent, Aikidoka, counsellor, gifted healer, for showing me how the shinobi heart should radiate the light of love and compassion and for guiding me to the bodhisattva path.

CONTENTS

Introduction

After disintegration comes reintegration. Many people fail to reach this stage. In my case it took fifteen years to find the right diagnosis and treatment for my illness. In those fifteen years I learned a lot about the mind and its workings. I couldn't see it then but I was learning skills for what I do now. After nearly twenty years' experience of fighting mental illness, I now consider myself to be an 'expert by experience'. This is also roughly the same amount of time I've been studying the martial arts: the way of Budo. At this fork in the road of my life, both paths seem to be merging to become one as I reach for the original purpose of both martial arts and mental healing:

psychic wholeness (enlightenment), while fulfilling my spiritual appetite at the same time.

I'm the man who put Humpty together again! Everybody needs mental health and wellbeing. I present to you my path through the darkness and delusion at the heart of mental suffering. I call it the Way of the Wayward Warrior.

'Respect the gods and buddhas, but do not depend on them', is what Miyamoto Musashi said in his *Book of Five Rings* (*Gorin No sho*). This is my *Book of Five Rings*.

The Way of the Wayward Warrior

FREEDOM

What does it mean to be truly free? Real freedom comes from within. It's a place inside us we can visit whenever we wish.

These days our freedom seems to be crumbling before our eyes. It can be hard to escape the constant psychological barrage of everyday life as well as the psychological cages that are created for us by the powers that be. Political spin, advertising, TV, radio, newspapers, schooling, religion, friends, family, parents and so on, all constantly bombard our psyches in an effort to bend us to their point of view. This is how cults gain members and politicians get you to vote for them. These are just some of our influences. It's strange to think that everything you know is only one truth, one way of looking at things. Truth is subjective, a matter of opinion.

There is one other person that cages us psychologically. It's you! At times, we are our own worst enemy, talking ourselves into dark corners and unhelpful beliefs that tie an anvil to the tail of our kites, crush our dreams and hopes and keep us in chains, living 'ordinary' lives.

We are the ones who do not actively challenge our thoughts and beliefs.

What is that little voice in your mind saying to you? What are you telling yourself? What have you been taught?

If you have problems you may find that you are stuck in one way of looking at things.

For instance, we may have a problem on our mind that won't go away, and we struggle with it for weeks, months on end. We drive ourselves into dark, black pits thinking, worrying about a particular problem or situation, turning it around in our heads. 'If only' comes into the picture, and we feel powerless and scared. Life, the elements, even God has it in for us.

We tire ourselves out with worry and then depression sets in, the classic negative spiral.

Have you ever felt doomed in this way? Cursed? Damned? Jinxed?

Whether you believe you can do something or not—you're right!

It's your belief that determines your reality.

If you believe you can, then you can. The opposite is also true.

> *'Work out your own salvation with diligence.'*
>
> —Buddha

Remember that no matter what you're thinking or what's on your mind, it is only a thought wave. When you really examine it, all it is is a little spark of energy flying through a couple of pounds of flesh and bone in your skull! You don't have to believe it.

There are other ways of looking at things.

Try to pull back to the centre and look for a more positive, rational truth. Can you see that it's only one way of looking at the situation? Can you see another way of looking at things? There are probably hundreds.

A good education shows you how to step aside and examine your own beliefs so that you don't make flawed assumptions based on conditioning.

This is real freedom, the freedom to take a step back and think about what you are saying to yourself or being told by others.

What are your beliefs? What are your influences saying to you? Are they being positive, do they nurture you? Do they encourage and support you? Or do they treat you badly and make you feel negative about things?

It would be very unfortunate to let others decide how you should feel.

Positive thought attracts positive energy.

The reverse is also true.

Watch what you think and what you take in. Be mindful of positivity. Stay free.

'If you don't eat your meat, you can't have any pudding!
How can you have any pudding if you don't eat your meat?'
—Pink Floyd

LUCK

I remember the World Cup song when I was little. It went something like:

> *'We have a dream,*
> *If dreams come true…'*

What I've learned about luck is that we make our own luck.

'If dreams come true…'? Indeed!

The Scottish World Cup squad were doomed to fail if that was their attitude.

They were like leaves blowing around the park, leaving it to forces outside themselves to magically blow them (or the ball) in the right direction.

They were really only booting the ball around in circles, not playing football.

If dreams come true… Well, did they make the dream come true?

Did they take positive action to bring about a win in the final—in other words, empowerment?

Or did they leave it up to the Gods and imaginary bogey-men to magically give them wings—disempowerment?

When we leave it all down to Lady Luck we throw away our

power to take positive action. Action that will make our dreams a reality. This is bad luck when you think about it. But if we rely on our own power to realise our dreams— self-reliance—we take positive action. This gives us more chance (luck) of attaining our dreams. Good luck!

Luck is inside us. It's the action we take to attain our goals.

We make our own luck.

PURPOSE

A purpose is something we all need to continue with our lives. To lose purpose is to lose the reason to live.

Many people blunder through life, blowing around like leaves on a breeze, hoping that maybe this week the big Lottery finger will come out of the sky and say 'IT'S YOU!'

Life feels dull and flat, and sometimes it seems there's no point getting out of bed in the morning. We learn little after we leave school, and are convinced by those around us that labouring, skivvying or the local biscuit factory is the best we can hope for in life. We start to believe our influences after a while, and past conditioning and negative reinforcement set in. We end up being just what everybody expected us to be.

Careers officers are a prime example of this kind of conditioning. 'Big boots, son? Skinheid? You'd make a great soldier! Ever thought about a career in the Army, son?'

You know the type. We don't have to listen to all this, though. We can decide for ourselves what we become, how we choose to live out our incarnation.

'If you always do what you've always done, you'll always get what you've always had.'

What would you be if you could not fail? What is your dream job, your ultimate lifestyle?

I took two weeks to come up with an answer to this question.

I believe that we're all here to carry out our life's mission. We all have a God-given role to play in the theatre of existence, to learn to achieve our purpose.

This gives our life meaning. To find our purpose we must look at what our time on earth has taught us. Think back over the span of your life. What lessons have you learned? If you look hard enough you may find there's a reason for all you've been through. Every situation you go through in life, no matter how hard, teaches you lessons. These lessons reveal your life's purpose.

Your destiny defines your purpose.

Have the same things been happening to you all your life? What is this showing you, what do you need to learn? What skills have you learned from life?

Maybe this is your calling. Learn from it. No matter how hard the lesson, you'll maybe find that it couldn't have been taught in any other way. In the end you may actually feel grateful for the lesson. Once we learn, we rarely get caught out again (at least not in the same way).

Obstacles instruct, not obstruct.

'We must walk through the darkness to find the light.'
—Graffiti

In my case I went through years of mental illness and I had to research ways to alleviate my symptoms. My beloved cat got sick, so I learned how to heal to help her. I also trained in the martial arts, and this gave me the spiritual toughness and psychological training to live through what I did. I'm not trying to be some sort of guru, just a mentally-ill guy who got his head together, and is passing on what helped him.

None of this has anything to do with the year 2000 or any of that New Age nonsense. Just practical lessons from the ancient ones, our ancestors. Very old technology.

My first book, *The One*, happened because I believed I could be a writer. I gave it a try, basically.

What do you believe you can do? What have you learned?

Keep a light at the end of the tunnel. You have a purpose. Everybody does.

Remember that no matter how painful the lessons you've had to learn, every event has a meaning in the grand scheme of things. All was meant to be for a reason.

RESPONSIBILITY

A lot of people who are ill go to their doctor and say 'Heal me, make me well.'

I have been guilty of this in the past. We expect the doctor to have a magic pill that will take away all our troubles. Life doesn't work like that. Maybe there is no quick cure for what ails you. A useful skill would be to meet the doctor half way. To do this we must communicate well and also learn about our own illness. I have been researching mental illness for nearly 20 years and I've only just scratched the surface.

When we think this way we realise that we have a re-sponsibility for our own illness as much as any doctor or psychiatrist. We are responsible for our own well-being more than anyone. Learn about your condition, become self-reliant. What you've been through has made you strong, stronger than you think. What you have learned has made you stronger and wiser than those who have never had many problems. You have knowledge that they don't have.

> *'Good timber is not grown with ease.*
> *The stronger the wind, the stronger the trees.'*
>
> —Anon

To those suffering like myself from mental illness, I would say that we have an obligation to act responsibly. Act as mad as you like, but try and keep a good heart throughout. You must be all you can be to inspire others who are just feeling their way. You cannot afford to let the side down as a mentally-ill person. Remember that every-thing you do in life has a consequence, an outcome. You could start by looking at personal development and edu-cating yourself. Try a college course. We could call this conscious evolution.

I strongly believe that if you could get it together you would have an edge over those who have had it easy in life. Carl Gustav Jung, the great psychologist and Sigmund Freud's student said that 'Neurosis can be used as a springboard towards personal growth and self-realisation.'

Rely on yourself and have faith in the universe. With this you can move mountains.

'The biggest room in the school is the room for improvement.'
—Anon

POTENTIAL

Everybody has potential. If only we really knew what we were capable of. The power remains locked at our core because we freeze and are afraid to take action. Fear is what holds us back, but so do our beliefs. Remember, if we think deep down that we can't do it, we won't.

Believe in yourself! If anyone with two arms, two legs and half a brain can do it then you can too. Even famous pop stars are just ordinary human beings when they knock off work. There is no super race of people, only folk like you and me. To get where they are, just do as they did. We only have a few years in this life to achieve our maximum potential, to be the most we can be. Better get on it now! The clock is ticking…

Aim high. Let your kite soar. Aim for the stars and you'll at least hit the moon!

'Om namu shivaya!'

—Sanskrit mantra

'Om namu shivaya!' (I bow before the possibilities that are in me!) Try repeating this mantra to yourself whenever you are in doubt about things.

If in doubt, a good approach is to bluff it until you can find a way. Fake it till you make it. You'll be very surprised at what you can do when the pressure's on.

Once you set your sights on a goal it's as if the power of the universe comes to your aid and conspires to bring your dreams to fruition. Have faith, the universe will provide…

All was meant to be.

NOW

Now is a special time. When you think about it, now is the only time that exists. When we look back at the past we can see that the past is dead and gone. Similarly, the future has not come to be yet, and when it does it'll be now again.

A lot of psychological problems have their roots in the past. We live in the past mulling over old wounds. But the past can't hurt us, it's gone. Stay in the now. Whenever you get down about the past, bring yourself back to the now. Come back to the now and change your situation.

Anxiety is mostly caused by worrying about the future. Again we are disconnected with the now. The future rarely turns out to be as bad as we imagine. When the time comes you'll be so wrapped up in what you are doing that it won't be as bad as you think. It would be a lot more helpful if you were to think about what you can do about it. You could make sure that it never happens the way you imagine by taking action now.

People sometimes put off things until later or when they feel better or such and such a time.

They procrastinate. To put things off till later just gives you more to worry about in the future, and you are throwing away your best chance of achievement. Later never comes. Do it now.

STIGMA

It's funny the amount of stigma I attracted as a mentally-ill person. People would belittle me because I didn't look at the world the same way they did. I was different, you see. It was all of them and then there was me. Sometimes people would even feel sorry enough for me to try and teach me how to think like them. Here I am 20 years later, teaching them how to think properly. I wonder if their way of looking at things really served them in life. I have found that a lot of the ones who were most vocal in stigmatising me are now wayward too…

They say that one in four people will suffer from mental illness at some time in their lives. One in a hundred will be schizophrenic. You should understand that to stigmatise someone with a mental illness is really hurting yourself. That could be your brother or sister, maybe even your mum or dad, God forbid. Always remember that there is a human being behind the illness. When I was ill my consciousness was intact. I was in there, seeing, feeling everything that was going on.

The important thing is to know that you can recover. I'm living proof.

There is always hope.

I can take a joke the same as the next man. But there's joking and there's joking. Never give in because of other people's ignorance.

'We are all fools at heart, but there are two types of fool in the world. Humorous fools and ignorant fools.'

—Dan Millman

DETERMINATION

The last thing I want to tell you about is determination. You must have the staying power to last the course. The harder you work for your goals, the luckier you'll get. You must persevere no matter what, and never allow yourself to be discouraged. Once you have set a goal you must bite like a bulldog, and no matter what anyone says you must not let go until you achieve it. It's not easy, but if it was then everybody would be millionaires and I would spend my time making babies with Anastacia, the heroine of my first book!

Remember that strength we talked about earlier. The strength that illness or adversity has made you develop. This is what makes you stand out from the crowd. Use it.

'Per ardua ad astra.'

—Latin proverb
('Through hardship to the stars.')

THE MIND: DEFINED

According to Sigmund Freud the mind is split into three parts, the Id, the Ego and the Super-ego. Freud saw these three component parts as competing for control.

THE ID (LATIN FOR 'IT')

This is our unconscious mind. It controls all the involuntary body functions and also our shadow side. The shadow side, as we'll see later, consists of all the unresolved emotions and problems that we deny and stick away in the back of our minds. All of this is stored in the unconscious.

The unconscious expresses itself through impulses like the desire to have sex, to eat when you are hungry and sleep when you are tired. The Id is concerned with instant gratification and is impulsive and childlike. The Id has little free will (thankfully) and absorbs whatever we programme into it (as in hypnosis) without question.

THE SUPER-EGO

The Super-ego, Freud felt, was the internal parent. It is the bit of us that keeps our morals and behaviour in check. The Super-ego is a bit like our parents telling us off when we're bad and praising us when we're good. The Super-ego is thought to develop around the age of six or seven, and is programmed into us by our early influences (parents, family, playmates, etc) as we grow up.

THE EGO

The Ego is the go-between. The Ego is responsible for collecting and sorting outside information and translating it into a version we can understand. As Geoff Thompson says in his book *Fear*, the Ego is like a bouncer who keeps out all the nasties that try to get into the pub (your unconscious mind). The Ego keeps out all the rubbish and useless stimulation in the universe.

Carl Jung was always at odds with his mentor Freud on this theory. Jung believed in another element of the self: consciousness or spirit. Jung had studied a lot of Eastern philosophy and he believed that life continued after physical death. He and Freud argued over this constantly. Freud warned Jung not to get lost in the 'occult' and it led to a falling out between the two. It is interesting to note that later Freud joined a society for paranormal exploration and also admitted to his students that his methods were outdated.

Personally, I think that although psychiatry has its place, it is based on hundred-year-old methods in which physical molecules and atoms (i.e., drugs and tablets) are used to fix mental (energetic) problems. This model is based on duality and does not take into account the holistic view. Also, I find that psychiatrists usually teach you how to concentrate on survival issues. This does not take the desires of the person into account and in effect, cuts them off from fulfilment. Like everybody else, mentally ill people have desires as well as needs, and to deny them is to settle for survival mode. We have a responsibility to swap neediness for compassion, to give out energy rather than taking it in.

THE MIND: A GUIDED TOUR

THE SUPER-EGO

The Super-ego is the internal parent. Think of a thing you did that you really regret. What do you feel guilty about?

This is the Super-ego at work. It shuns you with bad feelings when you do wrong but rewards you with warmth and energy when you do good.

THE EGO

Think of someone who really annoyed you by doing something to you. This is your Ego reacting. It's an inner feeling or voice that tells you that you don't like this person, can't stand them, or even want to punch them. The Ego is like our onboard computer. It interprets outside information and shows us it in a filtered, organised way that is understandable to us. The Ego can sometimes lie to us, showing us a distorted reality based on past conditioning.

THE ID

As we have seen, the Id is concerned with instant gratification. Think of someone you really had the hots for! This is the Id at work. Also when you are thirsty and want a drink right away. When you are hungry, tired, need to use the toilet, and so on.

THE MIND'S EYE

This part of the mind is the picture screen inside our minds, just above and between the eyes. This is where we imagine things in pictures.

EXERCISE

Picture in your mind an orange. Say the word orange to yourself in your mind. You can actually hear the word orange as you think it. This is your modality, your inner sense of hearing.

Now, still imagining the orange, peel off some of the skin, then lift the orange up to your nose (in your mind). Can you smell fresh orange? This is your modality of inner smell.

Now tear off a section of orange (mind your sticky hands!) and put the piece of orange in your mouth. You may start to salivate and actually taste orange. This is our inner sense of taste.

As you can see we not only have our five physical senses but also our inner senses. It is through these modalities that our mind communicates with our consciousness.

This was also your first lesson in visualisation. Remember, when visualising, use at least three of your inner senses or modalities to build up your picture. Picture yourself attaining your dreams, your goals. The more specific the detail you can picture, the more information you are sending to the subconscious mind to build with. The process is exactly the same as the orange-peeling visualisation.

I'll leave you with this to ponder: what actually sees the orange in your mind's eye? What tastes the orange? Smells it? Hears the word orange when you think it to yourself? For now let's just call it the Witness.

THE EFFECTS OF VARIOUS MENTAL CONDITIONS

Anxiety, panic, worry: the fear emotions come from our lower, emotional brain, the limbic system.

This system is a primitive part of the brain that comes from our reptilian ancestors, and it controls our fight-or-flight mechanism. This was useful to us back in the caveman days when we had to battle woolly mammoths and sabre-toothed tigers, but in the modern world it can limit us, and if not managed, can shorten our lifespan.

The upper brain (neo-cortex) registers a threat (real or imagined) and sends a message to the limbic system via the unconscious mind. The child-like unconscious can only follow orders and cannot think for itself, so it sends out a message to the body systems to be alert. It does this by way of the autonomic nervous system, in particular the sympathetic branch. This stimulates the adrenal glands and, Bingo!, you're in a panic.

Later, when the perceived threat has passed, we calm down naturally. Adrenaline secretion slows as the parasympathetic branch of the autonomic (involuntary) nervous system (otherwise known as the brakes!) kicks in, relaxing us. This rebalancing process is known as Homeostasis.

Homeostasis can be induced consciously in many different ways, including yoga, Qi gong and martial arts (especially Aikido and Tai Chi), as well as healing and some talking therapies. These are especially helpful when our fears are of an irrational nature, such as in anxiety and panic-attack sufferers. My personal belief is that panic sufferers have lost contact with the sacred in life. I have found (as a sufferer myself) that behind most people's panic attacks is a fear of dying and a fear of fear itself. When in the grips of a full-blown panic we think we're dying horribly… then our fear increases and we get more physical symptoms.

In the long term I would advise any anxiety sufferer to reconnect with spirit. (It may take you a while to fully realise what spirit is.) Ultimately you need to experience the sacred in life. This will bring about faith in the universe based on proof you've seen for yourself (i.e., not blind faith). When you learn to be rational again you will see that there really is nothing to worry about.

You'll find your shine again.

We'll look at many ways of inducing Homeostasis later, as well as finding a little faith!

DEPRESSION

Depression is a terrible mental condition that affects one in four of us in our lifetimes.

We all know how it feels to have 'the blues'. With depression, the mind and body cannot function properly because of the tremendous weight of problems pressing (depressing) on the consciousness. The sufferer can't function because of the mental anguish and pain they are experiencing, and they cannot see hope or any point in life. I myself have suffered from terrible bouts of depression—the sickness of waking up dreading another day ahead, wishing I would die to end the pain. This can be compounded with feelings of worry and anxiety. You feel 'scared to live but afraid to die' and life seems like a cruel punishment. Life on the whole should be a happy affair, though we will all have our ups and downs.

The way I see depression is that there's too much mental energy focused inwards, depressing the brain centres and consciousness and it needs to be released so the energy can flow freely again.

There are ways of treating this condition. We'll experience some of these later.

Know that the possibility of dropping darkness and heaviness from your life does exist. There is always hope.

ANGER

Anger is the fight side of 'fight or flight'. Again our lower reptilian brain has kicked in (caveman syndrome) and instead of fear we feel the urge to fight rather than running away. This was useful to our ancestors when hunting mammoths, but in modern times this primitive system is letting us down. We all need a bit of anger to carry us through, but it can spiral out of control leading to mental illness and ultimately physical illness, even an untimely death.

Anger never solves anything, and when we are trapped in repeated bouts of rage, problems occur because of our rash actions. We make a sow's ear out of a silk purse. Anger needs to be expressed or vented sometimes and not stifled, as this suppression can just build up like a pressure cooker and eventually explode.

This can lead to catastrophic results and again we're caught in the negative loop:

ANGER →   WRONG ACTION →   GUILT AND PAIN →

ANGER →   WRONG ACTION →   GUILT AND PAIN…

Anger is an energy, and can be used as a fuel if channelled safely into positive action.

Beware of displacing your anger. We may take it out on the wrong person because someone cut us up on the road on the drive to work. We get home and moan at the wife that we've had a bad day. The kids are running about making a racket and we snap at them. The wife steps in to defend them and we end up rowing with her... all because someone cut us up in the car this morning. It's much better to vent your anger safely and healthily.

We'll look more at anger later.

SCHIZOPHRENIA / VOICE-HEARING

Schizophrenia is a serious illness of the mind and has nothing to do with split personalities. The sufferer hears voices and may see or feel things that are not physically there. The theory is that the conscious filter (a bit like a bouncer on a pub door) is worn down to such an extent that all the rubbish floating around the universe (troublemakers!) can gain direct access to your unconscious mind (the pub). This creates the bizarre symptoms the sufferer experiences, and it is thought that neurotransmitters in the brain are responsible. In schizophrenia the neurotransmitter dopamine is thought to be a major factor.

The voices are very intelligent and can bring helpful as well as harmful messages. The voices can be a signal of more serious problems deep in the psyche.

A good technique I have used is called 'focusing'. I look at the effect of the voices' messages in my mind. For instance, how do the voices make me feel? Guilty? Then I work on my conditioned guilt patterns. Do they make me feel scared? If so, I work on handling fear. And so on until I resolve all my problems with voices. If you suffer from voice-hearing, hopefully this will quiet them down a bit for you too.

It is interesting to note that the neurotransmitter dopamine is also secreted by the adrenal glands during fight-or-flight response. This may point to a trigger for schizophrenia, but the cause is thought to be genetic. Western medicine cannot cure this condition yet, but many have been helped by Chinese medicine. There is always hope.

BEREAVEMENT / SUICIDE

Suicide is different from other deaths. It tears apart those left behind and destroys relationships forever. In 1997 my mother Christine took her own life aged 47. It devastated me and tore my family apart. What I learned about suicide is that the person must feel so much pain that the only way out (they think) is to die. I have been through this myself when I was psychotic. I made serious attempts to take my own life several times. Thankfully I lived. There is always hope while you still breathe. My mother didn't make it, though. I learned that the survivors go through a series of emotional stages similar to those described by Elizabeth Kübler-Ross in *On Death and Dying.*

The five stages I went through were:

1. *Numbness and disbelief.*
At first there was a complete blankness, an emotional void, a numbness. I couldn't believe she was gone.

2. *Pining.*
This is the heartbreaking part. You miss the person so much you feel like your heart has been torn from your chest. I have never missed someone so much in my life.

3. *Depression / anger.*
In this stage you slip down into a depressed state as you try to come to terms with your loss and all that entails. You may go through bouts of anger and rage about why your loved one has been taken away from

you, and you may even feel angry at the person that died. This is natural, don't feel guilty about it.

4. *Acceptance.*

Eventually you begin to accept your loss. You come to terms with the person's absence and you begin to build a new life, a new normality without your loved one.

You may slip back periodically to the depressed state, but at this stage you can also remember the good times you had with the person.

5. *Recovery.*

This is the stage where you get yourself back together and start to get on with your life. You may still cry from time to time about the person, but this stage entails letting go of the past and living with the new reality. The pain is mostly over (never completely) and time puts distance between you and the hurt.

A SOLUTION?

A holistic experiment:

Imagine you could take all the energy you waste on 'going mad' (or just being stressed) and channel it into your life's goals, your dreams. You could design your own future if you think about it…

I have in the past 19, almost 20 years, learned that Western medicine mostly treats a symptom of illness and not the cause. In the East they believe we should attack the root of illness. The cause, not the symptom. In Western medicine the balance of neurotransmitters in the brain is a factor in most mental illness. The neurotransmitters can be influenced negatively (as in stress or a life event) so why not positively? Also, in Eastern thought a mental illness is a disease of the heart/mind (not heart disease!). This is where our thoughts and emotions come in. This book, describing the Way of the Wayward Warrior, is designed with this in mind, body and spirit. The result I want for you is perfection. To be all you were meant to be. I want you to have harmony, coherence at all levels.

The purpose of the Way is to heal and strengthen the body, to gain control of and quiet the mind and to realise and radiate the spirit. Conscious evolution.

We begin as a caterpillar and enter the cocoon. Eventually a beautiful butterfly emerges in all its glory…

Rebirth, in a way.

My Story

I was born in 1970 and brought up in Muirhouse, Edinburgh. At the age of 17 I started to suffer from anxiety and panic attacks after experimenting with hallucinogenic drugs. My mind was scrambled after one trip too many. Repeated trips to the doctor would reveal nothing. It was 'all in my head, psychosomatic', they'd pronounce. I was sent for talking therapy after talking therapy for anger, depression, anxiety, panic, agoraphobia. These helped to some extent, but I felt like the little Dutch boy with his finger in the dyke, holding back the flood. I got by for a while with exercise (cycling) but every time I fixed a leak the energy would burst out somewhere else.

Around this time I took up martial arts. I studied Genbukan Ninpo (Ninjutsu) under sensei James Wright for around six years, as well as other bits and pieces from Aikido and other arts. This turned into a study of Budo (warrior ways) and other Eastern philosophies, and I have continued my training to the present day.

Back to the illness. In 1997 I woke up one morning to find my mother dead. She'd committed suicide after a long depression, aged only 47. I was devastated. My world, my family, everything blew apart. I enrolled in college in an effort to escape my world, to learn my way out of my predicament. I studied communications, philosophy, psychology and student support, which introduced me to different learning methods. My illness started to worsen. I began to believe everybody in college was a threat to me. I started to become paranoid. I had to drop out of college after a particularly bad panic attack.

I began to withdraw from life. I shunned all my so-called friends, unplugged my phone and refused to answer the door—sometimes even to family. I started to read and study self-help and self-improvement books. I'd read a book on legendary 16th-century sword master Miyamoto Musashi. Musashi had been a wild youth (like myself) in feudal Japan who'd got himself into so much trouble that the locals hunted him down like an animal. He was captured by Samurai who wanted to crucify or behead him as the mad dog he was. Takuan, a local monk, took pity on poor Musashi and pleaded with the local lords to let him punish Musashi as he saw fit. The lords agreed, and Takuan put Musashi in the top room of a haunted castle with nothing but books for company and locked the door. Musashi never saw a soul for four years, but after the time elapsed the door to the room was opened and a new Musashi came out. Musashi dropped to his knees and thanked Takuan for setting him free, taming the wild beast he'd become.

Musashi fought over a hundred documented duels in his lifetime which he dedicated to mastery of swordsmanship. He died of old age after writing his strategy book *Gorin No Sho*, or *Book of Five Rings*. His grave site is a place of pilgrimage even today.

After reading this story I began to wonder what Musashi could possibly have learned to change him so much. I had the haunted castle and a library full of books at the end of my road, so I thought I'd do the same and lock myself away with books. I read obsessively, day and night. Without realising it I grew more and more paranoid. My illness worsened slowly but constantly, and I began to lose touch with reality. All the while I studied. Books on self-help, self-improvement, health and healing, martial arts, diet, the list went on. Then one day my world caved in. After years of mental illness I woke up one morning and decided life wasn't worth living. I took an over-dose of my medication and lay down to die.

I awoke, angry that I was still alive. It was around then I began to see things, have strange thoughts and hear voices. I started to follow the wind that I believed had been sent to guide me around the streets of Edinburgh on a mission for Scotland.

> *'Left broken,*
> *Empty and despaired,*
> *On a breeze,*
> *Can't find air.'*
>
> —Anastacia

To cut a long story short I ended up in the Royal Edin-burgh Hospital for four months on a Section 18, i.e. I was compulsorily detained. I was finally given the diagnosis of schizophrenia in September 2001. After I got out of hospital I decided I wanted to write about what had happened to me. It was so amazing I just had to show somebody. I'd jotted down mind maps (little thought bubbles with key words written in them) of my experiences of schizophrenia, and these reminded me of each episode. I sat down to write my first book *The One*. (I started to type with two fingers at first. I had to teach myself to type and use a computer!) Six months later I'd completed the first draft. I sent it away to publishers, but it came back with knock back after knock back. I showed my aunt who showed it to her friend Quintin Jardine, the crime writer, and he was impressed, so impressed he showed it to a publisher friend at Mercat Press. They made me an offer and the book was published less than two years after I got out of hospital. I believe it was my iron determination that got me through, and hard work. Talent never came into it much.

#

The rest of the Way is divided into five parts (Elements). The five Elements are an ancient metaphysical way of looking at the world. I first learned of them through my martial art, but they've been around forever. I think the simplicity of the system is what attracts me the most, but also the complexity of the subject. In the beginning there was nothing, only the source. The emptiness became charged with two polarities, which formed into atoms. The particles became nebulous and formed into gases. The gases combusted and water began to condense, then evaporate, leaving solid matter. Profound, I'm sure you'll agree.

The Elements

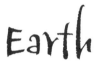

Earth

(Body Arts)

CHI BALL

Rub your hands together briskly to warm them and raise the chi. *(Chi is the energy of the universe, and will be described in more detail in the Fire chapter.)* Relax—chi is easy. Don't use too much effort.

Place your hands together as if in prayer and then gently and slowly let them part (around six inches). Try to feel the energy between your two hands. You may feel heat or a sense of magnetism, a fluffy feeling between your hands. Form this energy into a ball. See how far you can part your hands and still feel the chi. Play around with the chi ball. You may wash your face with the chi, paying particular attention to the area around the eyeballs. You may feel the chi penetrating your eye sockets and gently warming them. Bring your hands back to the prayer position (hands together) in front of your chest to end the exercise. Practice this exercise to feel the chi whenever you get a spare minute and you'll develop chi sensitivity. We'll be working with this energy a lot in later exercises.

THREE INTENTFUL CORRECTIONS

Be aware of the three corrections throughout the day. The three corrections are a way of removing obstacles that inhibit chi flow in the body. They are:

1. *Posture*: Align the head, back and hips. Relax. The physiology affects the mind.

2. *Mind*: Empty your mind of all thoughts (this takes practice, and we will return to this in the next chapter) or visualise the flow of chi with the breath. This is thinking of one thing and you should not let in any other thoughts that interrupt you.

3. *Breath*: Breathe slowly and deeply, in and out of the abdomen (*hara*). Relax. *Never force the breath*.

These three checks themselves can lead to a state of harmony and calm. Make them a habit and keep your head up. (Never look at the floor when dealing with people.)

ZHAN ZHUANG (STANDING LIKE A TREE)
(See illustrations on p. 45)

To begin, hold each posture for 1 minute.

Remember to clear the mind, straighten posture and breathe from the abdomen.

Visualise energy flowing in as you breathe in.

Visualise stagnant and stale energy (illness) flowing out on exhalation.

RELAXATION

Make sure you will not be disturbed for around 20 minutes and maybe unplug the phone.

Lie down on your bed or couch and loosen any tight clothing.

Take a deep breath and hold it. When the breath needs to come out, gently release it and let your eyes fall closed.

Relax, let go. Make sure your teeth are not clenched together and relax your jaw.

Start with your scalp muscles. Relax. Feel the tension ease out of the scalp and flow down to your forehead.

Relax and let go.

Relax your forehead in just the same way. Feel the tension go and relax.

Now think about your eyes. Relax your eyes. There are lots of small muscles around your eyes, relax these muscles. Let your eyelids feel heavy and relaxed.

Again relax your jaw and all your facial muscles.

Let this feeling spread down to your neck. Your head is starting to feel heavy as you relax your neck. Let go. Relax.

Let go of any tension in your shoulders and down through the muscles in your arms. Relax right down to the tips of your fingers. Let go.

Now think about the trunk part of your body. Relax. Let all the tension melt away from the trunk part of your body. Letting go…

Let the feeling of relaxation spread down through the muscles in your legs. Down through the muscles of your thighs and calves, all the way to the very tips of your toes.

Relax, let go, drift…

You may wish to speak this script into a tape recorder to listen to as you relax.

ZHAN ZHUANG (STANDING LIKE A TREE)

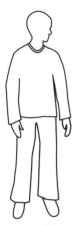

Wu chi

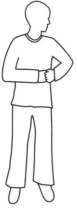

Holding ball to chest

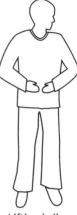

Lifting belly

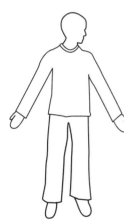

Standing in a stream

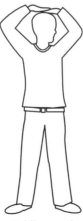

Holding up sky (palms up)

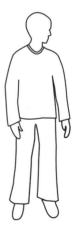

End in wu chi

HARA (THE NAVEL)

If you ever feel nervous (or suffer from anxiety), then you need to ground yourself.

1. Put your hand on your hara (1 inch below the belly button).

2. Put your mind in your hara (don't think too much about how to do it, just put your concentration there).

3. Breathe in through the nose and out through the mouth.

4. Try to get a feeling of heaviness, a sinking-into-the-ground sort of feeling.

This exercise comes from the martial art of Aikido. It is used to control fear.

MAKKO HO

Try these stretching exercises (*see illustrations, opposite*). They were specifically created by a Shiatsu practitioner called Mr Makko and are used to unblock the chi pathways in the body and organ channels.

MAKKO HO

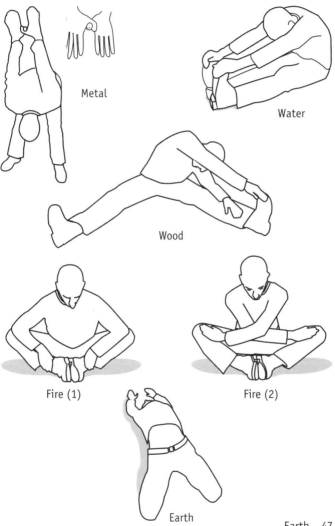

Metal

Water

Wood

Fire (1)

Fire (2)

Earth

Water
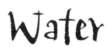

(Mind Boxing)

'A distorted mind acts to create a distorted reality resulting in suffering.'
    —Thich Nhat Hahn

PERSONAL CLARITY

Practise the three exercises on the following pages to train the mental process. Try to become proficient at each one before moving on to the next one. Build up to 10 minutes a day.

1. BREATH COUNTING

No-mind state can be hard to achieve. We start the process of mind training by focusing the mind on one activity. This is known as mindfulness.

Go into meditation and quiet the mind. When the stream of thoughts begins to subside, start to focus on your breathing. Do not try to control the breath, simply watch the rise and fall of your abdomen.

As you breathe in, count 1.

Watch your abdomen fall as you breathe out.

Breathe in again and count 2.

And so on until you've breathed in and out nine times.

Then start to count from 1 again.

Keep on counting your breaths from 1 to 9 as long as you can (at least 5 to 10 minutes).

You may become distracted and find yourself counting 10, 11, 12…

Just start counting from 1 again.

1 to 9…

2. GAME OF STONES

This exercise is to discipline the mind and turn down the volume of your racing thoughts.

Pick up a pebble or small object (natural objects are best) and go into meditation.

When you've quietened the stream of thoughts, open your eyes and observe your pebble.

Do not allow yourself to think in words or pictures, just observe the pebble in your hand.

Try to observe every minute detail of your pebble without thinking in words. (This takes a lot of effort at first—don't give up!)

Try to feel the pebble, absorb the characteristics of its texture, colour, abrasiveness, smoothness.

Repeat the same exercise again and again with the same pebble. Try to notice something new each time as you go to deeper and deeper levels of peace.

This exercise will bore you to tears at first. It can be frustrating, I know. That is the point of it. To train the mind to do as you tell it, not the other way around.

Beyond boredom lies real achievement. Persevere.

3. ONE-POINTEDNESS

Focus

Sit cross-legged or in a chair, straight-backed, and go into meditation. When you calm the stream of thoughts (this should be easier now after last week's exercise) open your eyes and stare at your chosen spot.

Don't picture anything and don't think in words, just simply stare.

After a while you may find yourself daydreaming. Empty your mind again and focus on your chosen spot. Above all—RELAX!

Good focus points for this exercise are: a lit candle, a tack in the wall, a bonsai tree. Even a mark on the ceiling would do.

This exercise should be done gently and not forced in any way. Mental training requires a lot of effort and can be harder than physical training.

You may find this the hardest exercise you've ever done. Persevere. Boredom and frustration will give way to peace, clarity, laser-like focus and concentration.

'Who looks outside, dreams; who looks inside, awakens.'
— Carl Gustav Jung

QI GONG
BUDDHA BELLY BREATHING

This exercise flushes the brain and clears toxins from the body. It pumps the cells (including the brain) full of nutrient-enriched blood, water and oxygen, and stores chi in the abdomen. It is a cleansing breath.

Breathe in through the nose for the count of 6.

Breathe in to the hara (an inch below the belly button).

Hold for one, one thousand, two, one thousand, three, one thousand.

Breathe out through the mouth for 6.

Hold for one, one thousand, two, one thousand, three, one thousand.

Repeat 6 to 10 times.

As you breathe in, visualise good chi flowing in through your nose and down your front to your abdomen.

As you breathe out, visualise stagnant chi (your illness or stress), toxic chi and disturbed chi flowing from your mouth.

ZHAN ZHUANG 2

Go back to the standing like a tree exercise from the Earth chapter (pp. 43, 45).

Do the exercises again but this time hold each posture for 2 minutes and count your breaths 1-9 as you learned earlier. The game is to focus on keeping the mind counting while ignoring the body.

The whole set of exercises should take 12 minutes.

'All the trees, all the grass is for the Emperor.
Where can demons live?'

— Samurai saying

'Heaven's gates won't hold me,
I'll saw those suckers down
Laughing loud at your locks,
When they hit the ground'

— Stone Roses.

BUTTERFLY BREATH

The next time you have a pain take a few deep breaths and relax.

As you breathe into the abdomen visualise yourself taking in and storing good chi in the *hara* (an inch below the navel).

As you breathe out, direct a stream of chi with your mind to the source of the pain.

Visualise good chi flowing from your hara to the pain site as you breathe out.

Do this for a few minutes and you should find the pain dispersing.

JOSHIN KOKYU HO:
CLEARING THE MIND/EXPANDING PRESENCE

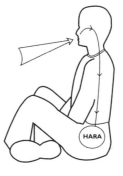

1. BREATHE IN:
Breathe in through the nose and down into the hara.

2. BREATHE OUT:
Breathe out through the nose and imagine inflating a protective bubble.

SPANKING THE MONKEY

Mindfulness of thought. Detachment from the ego.

The mind in most people is unruly. Buddha likened the mind to a monkey swinging from branch to branch. Another way it resembles a monkey is that it has a mischievous nature and it chatters like a monkey in a tree despite our efforts to cease thinking.

The Chinese likened the mind to wild horses that need breaking in. The Japanese see the mind as a wild tiger, dangerous when left to roam of its own free will.

The mischievous monkey has a trick that it can play on most of us too. You see, every time the monkey opens his gibbering mouth he spits out an A.N.T.

Automatic

Negative

Thought

These are automatic thoughts of a negative type that the monkey sneaks in to keep us feeling bad. When we feel bad we are under the monkey's spell. He controls us in that moment.

The monkey is a liar as you will eventually see. His game is to keep us under his A.N.T. spell so he can tease us with his chatter.

The monkey is really our Ego.

A.N.T.s are the random thoughts that flit through our untrained minds.

Watch your mind thinking. What are you thinking? What are you saying to yourself?

Just because we think something doesn't make it true. There are other ways of looking at the situation. If you analyse what you are saying to yourself you may actually see that it's not true. It's only the (negative, irrational) way we were looking at things.

Don't let A.N.T.s slip through. Look for a more positive, rational truth.

A practice known as Cognitive Behaviour Therapy (CBT) can be used to combat A.N.T.s. Fill in the blank CBT sheets at the back of this book. Add an entry every time you feel bad. Write down what you are saying (what the monkey is saying) to yourself when you feel bad.

Look for a more positive, rational way of looking at things and write this in the next box.

Do this exercise over the next few weeks so you can gradually detach from the monkey mind and change your habits of Automatic Negative Thinking.

'There's a monkey in the family,
It was trained by Adam and Eve.
It was sold to your great-great grandpa and grandma
And decided it wouldn't leave.'

—Happy Mondays

DEMON CRUSHING

Emotions derive from our early influences and are conditioned into us (often combined with a clout!) As we explore the emotions, you may come to see that a lot of what I would call inappropriate emotion comes from basic lies that we tell ourselves. Our early influences passed them on to us before we were six, and we've kept them on our hard drives ever since. Your parents in turn probably had all this whacked into them too.

'Mother, should I build a wall?'

—Pink Floyd

When we examine these lies under the light of awareness, it's like shining a torch on a shadow—literally our shadow side! Emotions can be at the root of psychiatric illness as well as a constant stress to the body and mind of the person suffering.

If left unchecked, these wild tigers can create chaos in your life and can develop into physical and/or mental symptoms.

The five emotions are:

> Anger
>
> Fear
>
> Guilt
>
> Sorrow (grief)
>
> Worry

ANGER

The trick with this volatile emotion is not to jump the gun in your thinking. Before you explode with rage there is a thought wave. This is usually an A.N.T. You don't know for sure that the person annoying you is being contemptuous or trying to wind you up. When we get angry in this way we tend to make assumptions that are not based in truth. We go with our angry thoughts and end up lashing out over a misunderstanding. Also, we get angry through frustration when we feel disempowered. We flare up to redress the balance of energy in the conflict, to regain control of the situation. Anger is a control issue.

FEAR

Fear is the emotion of flight. You want to get yourself out of harm's way. At the origin of most fears is a thought wave.

You tell yourself that you can't handle the situation you are experiencing. This goes straight to your unconscious mind (which is childlike and can only follow orders) and it alerts the body systems to secrete adrenaline and other chemicals. You panic and run or feel ill. To fight fear you must catch the thought and override it. Tell yourself 'I can handle this'. The trick is to invite more of the fear feelings in while confronting the stressor. This is how exposure therapy works. If you invite it in the fear backs off. You defeat the monkey mind. No bananas tonight for the cheeky chump! Do this intermittently so as to get plenty of rest between battles. You can win this war! I'm living proof.

GUILT

This is one bad baby! Your Super-ego starts to punish you for transgressions, real and imagined. The thing with guilt is, IT'S A LIE!

Yes, this is one of those old nuggets of family wisdom passed down through the generations to control you. You see, guilt is just a porky pie when you get to the bottom of it. Nothing really means anything other than the meaning you (or someone else) gives it. Usually guilt is conditioned into us around age six or seven by our influences.

We are told we are bad by someone else when we do something that displeases them. Really it's just a method of controlling you.

Eventually we try harder to please and feel good about ourselves when we do. But we also punish ourselves with conscience when we do what we were told is bad. Guilt is just a habit programmed into us. Why should you let someone else decide how you feel about yourself and your past actions? Sometimes we just make mistakes. We don't really mean anything bad. We did the best with the learning we had at the time. Past mistakes don't make us bad people. And we can't please everybody all the time. Some people just can't be pleased so it's futile even to try.

Your heart should decide if something is right or wrong. Ask your heart.

SORROW

Otherwise known as depression or sadness. The thing with sadness, as with fear, is to catch the thoughts. The monkey mind may be playing tricks on us again if we're caught in a loop of automatic negative thinking. Yes, it's those darned A.N.T.s again. Sometimes we don't need to fight the blues. Just accept how you feel and experience it. This vents the system a bit and hopefully we get through sorrow by accepting it. If you tackle the negative thoughts that make you feel sad you will always look on the bright side.

Learn to think positively (and rationally) and this will get you through sadness. Also, have a good cry! This releases chemicals that cause depression, and flushes out emotional energy and blockages. Your tears contain toxic matter. Go have a bawl!

WORRY

Worry is when (in our subconscious) we try to predict future outcomes. We look ahead and decide that we can't handle it. What you need to do in the long run is learn to have faith. Trust (with practice) that the universe, nature, God, whatever, will come to your aid once you set a goal. Tell yourself that no matter what happens, 'I can handle this.' You need to experience the sacred and spiritual in life to see with your own senses that really there is nothing to worry about. The whole universe is on your side! Don't let those A.N.T.s get the better of you. Look forward (after imagining the worst-case scenario) and visualise a happy outcome. Then go about making sure that the future never happens the way you fear. Take positive action now. Eventually you will learn to have faith and guide yourself to your desired goals.

#

Work on each emotion one at a time. They may take a while to shift, so keep a journal so you know where you are. Remember that sometimes your emotions are justified and appropriate. At such times it is okay to express them. Honest communication is the best way to express your anger.

> '*He who fights with monsters might take care lest he thereby become a monster.*'
>
> —Friedrich Nietzsche

Fire

(Personal Energy)

ENERGY

Qi (chi) has many names in different cultures across the world. The Indians call it 'prana', the Japanese call it 'ki', Polynesians 'mana', Native Americans 'the great spirit' and Christians speak of Light.

It was the study of alchemists in ancient Europe, high priests in ancient Egypt (who called it 'ka'), and ether was the name given to the pure clean mountain air breathed by the Olympians in ancient Greece. Even science has its equivalents; in modern times it has been called the 'quantum field', and the 'Higgs field'.

Wilhelm Reich, the famous cloudbusting scientist named it 'orgone energy', Carl Gustav Jung the 'collective unconscious'. Hans Mesmer, the father of hypnosis, referred to it as 'animal magnetism', while Albert Einstein talked about a 'cosmological constant'.

When we look up at the sky most of us see only emptiness.

Buddhist and Taoist Qi gong (or Chi kung) masters look up at the sky and see the chi field or 'dao'. They have recognised the Qi field for thousands of years, while modern physicists have only in the last century or so begun to understand the quantum field. The chi field or quantum field has been found to be composed of countless packets and waves of energy which either act independently or in unison, like one giant, conscious particle. In quantum physics these are studied as subatomic particles. In Qi gong we study chi which is composed of such particles and waves. To become one with the field—which is really the whole universe—is to become Enlightened.

The Tibetans call this field the 'void', and the Buddhists 'the Buddha nature'.

Christianity refers to this 'intelligence' above as the Kingdom of God or Heaven, and Jews call the energy 'Rauch'.

Hindus call this Brahman, and in Islam Moslems teach this as a return to God or the Realisation of God.

As you will see, all religions seem to teach the same concepts, so to think in this way will not go against anyone's religious beliefs. It may even enhance them. To become one with the universe and meet what people call God is really the highest human endeavour. It makes you wonder why all the fighting between religions in the world goes on. Is this really what the one creator of the universe would want in his/her name?

We are all one.

Modern scientists have only in the last century or so begun to view the universe as one all-inclusive totality, a truth the ninja knew for a thousand years. Nothing and no one is really separate. We are all one. Even modern science has proved that we are all interconnected. This is an expression of chi, the energy of the universe. Like a fish swims in water, humans swim in chi. This view has been held since prehistory in most cultures, including our own. We call the full realisation of this knowledge enlightenment or sainthood—psychic wholeness. This is truly to see the oneness in everything, a deep realisation, and to some, a union with God.

'The sun will shine on you again.
A bell will ring inside your head,
and all will be brand new.'

—Oasis

SEEING CHI

To see chi or cosmic, universal energy, lie down and look up at the blue sky on a sunny day.

Relax your gaze and just stare a while. After a time you may begin to see little blobs of transparent energy whizzing around in the sky in front of your eyes.

The little blobs or pin-points of energy spin and flit around in the blue. This is chi. This is the energy we take in when we do qigong. This is universal life-force energy. You may find the little spots of energy in the sky whizz about faster on a sunny day than on a cloudy one.

CHANNEL YOUR ENERGY

Imagine you could take all the effort and energy you waste on 'going mad' or being stressed and channel it into your dreams, your life goals, your purpose.

Think of all the time you've wasted in your life being ill and feeling bad. All the time wasted trying to get back to 'normal', trying to be the way you used to be.

All of this took energy. Think of how you waste energy on a daily basis.

If you could get it together and channel this energy into your goals then it would be a fuel.

If you are an angry person, then this energy could be channelled too. This energy could set you ahead of the pack. It is your 'edge'.

MANIFESTING

Learn the power of I.G.T.V.A.

Intent

Goals

Thoughts

Visualisation

Action

Intent. The intention to do something is all you need. No maybes. If anyone with two arms and two legs can do something then you can too. Use them as a model. Do as they did.

Goals. Set a goal to aim for. If you don't have a goal to aim at you're not playing football, are you?

Thoughts. Get the thought right. Tell yourself 'I CAN

DO IT!' Look for excuses to succeed, not excuses to fail.

Visualisation. Go to the pictures in your head. Daydream about achieving your goal. Use at least three inner senses out of five to build your visualisation as in the orange exercise (*see p. 21*). This gives the unconscious mind more detail to work with. Mental rehearsal, if you like.

Action. If you don't take action then you are just dreaming. Taking action makes it physical. Do something every day to bring yourself closer to your dream. Start with something you can do NOW!

> *'You don't need eyes to see, you need vision.'*
> —Faithless

MAP FROM B TO A

To make a map, just ask yourself what you would need to learn to achieve your goal.

For example, I wanted to write books.

To be a writer I needed to get a book published. To get a book published I needed to write one. To write one I needed to learn how to write. To learn to write I needed to learn how to use a computer. To learn to use a computer I needed to get one and so on, until I got it down to something I could do that very moment to start off on my road to being a writer.

This is how a map from B to A is drawn. Just follow it. It's like baking a cake. Easy as that, follow the recipe.

OUTCOMES

Remember that whatever you do there will be an outcome. Most people leave the outcome to chance. Whatever happens to them, happens. This is a bit like a leaf blowing around in the wind. If you take charge now, take positive action, then you can guide yourself to the desired outcome. This is like a ship that uses a rudder to guide itself to its destination, its outcome. Design your own future, now! Steer your ship out of the harbour and navigate to your destination!

(You may find it helpful to fill in the Contract on the following page.)

CONTRACT

I PROMISE TO MYSELF that I will do my very best to

....

starting right now.

I will not deviate from the path I set myself until I

achieve my desired outcome.

I will research and look for excuses to succeed, not

excuses to fail.

I will achieve this goal before

....

Signed

....

Date

....

QIGONG: INTERNAL ALCHEMY

Sit cross-legged and take a few deep breaths.

Focus on the breath and breathe into the abdomen.

In nature water sinks. Fire burns upwards, it rises.

In alchemy we reverse the process.

As you breathe in, direct the chi from your abdomen to your sternum.

This is water rising.

As you breathe out, direct the chi from your head to your sternum.

This is fire descending.

Visualise.

The vapour of the fire and water collects in the heart/mind.

This is *xin*, an elixir for the mind.

LAUGHING BUDDHA

Take a couple of deep breaths and let your eyes fall closed on the out breath.

Think of a time when something funny happened or a happy time in your life. Remember your inner smile: let the smile come from deep within you, spreading joy throughout your whole being, chasing any negativity out.

You should find a smile has come to your face, or even a giggle!

NINNIKU SEISHIN

When dealing with negative people we usually find our-selves getting angry and frustrated. When this happens on a global scale we end up in wars and all sorts of suffering ensues. That is because most people react instinctively and jump to the first (automatic, negative) thought that comes into their heads when they feel insulted. There is another more productive way to deal with such confrontations, how-ever. We can choose to laugh! When we see the humour in a situation we can laugh at almost anything. We use joy to beat our enemy. The more they flare up, the more we laugh it off and refuse to be manipulated into an angry response. This totally disempowers an opponent who will find no chink in your armour to pry at.

Another good way to deal with angry, irate people is to burst into song! This totally throws them off, they think you're mad and give up, most unsettled!

This type of attitude is called 'Ninniku Seishin'.

Cultivate this kind of heart, refuse to be knocked out of your happy frame of mind.

'Or the love you bring,
won't mean a thing,
unless you sing,
Sing, sing, sing.'

—Travis

Wind

(Compassionate Heart)

'To show mercy and have a tender heart is to be truly human.'

—Toshitsugu Takamatsu, Ninja Grandmaster

THE HEART

The organ we call the heart is a complex device thought of as no more than a crude pump in Western medicine. The Oriental view however is more in line with our own forefathers' beliefs about the heart, and modern science is just beginning to catch on.

Most of us will have heard the saying 'don't let your heart rule your head', but I find that the big mistake we make in the human race is that *we let our heads rule our hearts*.

In modern society we are taught that the brain is the centre of thought, so we think in our heads. Our teachers, parents and peers tell us to 'Think!', 'Use your head!', 'Apply your brain!'

We literally get this lie, this half-truth, battered into us. We are brainwashed at school from a young age to believe only in what we see (logic and science, which deals in only physical proof). Is it any wonder we end up with problems in later life?

In the East and historically in the West we thought with an equal measure of head and heart. This creates a balanced view of life which is based on compassion and contemplation, passion and desire in equal measure. Our hearts are the centre of our feelings and to deny this is to cut ourselves off from what we feel. The problems in the world are mostly caused by living only in the head and having no feelings. We become inhuman and commit atrocities.

'Love is the key.'
—The Charlatans

The love I speak of is not some vague, metaphysical power, nor is it the cheesy puppy love we experience in adolescence. I'm not suggesting we walk around blissed-out, kidding on we're Jesus. Care-bears and happy-clappers need not apply! Love is an energy, just like electricity. Or chi, for that matter. Chi that is made in the heart. When we feel this energy for another person it causes many positive changes in the body and mind, and this is what we crave when we are 'in love' with someone. Just to have a happy respect for another human being, or even a pet, is a form of love. I lived alone with my cat Puddin for 9 years. I never had such a loyal friend. She taught me the meaning of unconditional love.

Can you imagine the parties we could have if everyone concentrated on broadcasting love and respect for each other? When I was growing up it was this energy that held my whole community together, even though I come from one of the roughest estates in Edinburgh. It's what makes a family a family, and when we lack this energy in our lives we are in our blackest moments. Look at any human being and you can at the very least love or appreciate them for just being human like you. Show a little love if you want love. Like attracts like. Send out a loving vibe to all you encounter.

If we all thought this way things would run a lot more harmoniously in this world.

Love is the law!

If in doubt ask your heart. Use it to guide you like a compass. What is done in love can't go far wrong.

XIN

This balance of heart and head in Chinese medicine is called xin, the heart/mind elixir. Xin leads to harmony, balance of heart and head or *coherence* as it is called in the west. Coherence is seen as the balance of the emotional (limbic) brain and heart rhythm. When our lower emotional brain is out of synch with our heart rhythm we are in the chaos rhythm. Usually this means we are stressed or depressed about something. In this state our heart and other organs labour and are out of synch with each other. Over time this can lead to premature ageing and ill-health, wear and tear on the body. We are not running at optimal function in this state.

In the coherent state, however, we synchronise heart and head through the breath. This leads to increased function of body and organs as our self-healing mechanisms are triggered. We may come out of our depression and get a feeling of well-being as well as enhanced intuition. We achieve a balance. This is what we experience when we are in the *flow*.

The heart guides us to what we desire, and the brain (mind) gets us there as efficiently as possible. We attain our goals leading to self-fulfilment.

> *'One love,*
> *One heart,*
> *Let's get together*
> *And feel alright.'*
>
> —Bob Marley

BUDDHA'S SMILE

Start to practice loving someone or something.

1. Put your right hand on your heart and feel your heart beat.
2. Take your hand off and just feel your heart beating.
3. Think of the person you love (or have loved) most in the world. Picture them in your mind.
4. Send them a big cuddle as you let the feeling of love flow from your heart.

You can practice on your partner, your child, a pet, even a beautiful plant.

It takes a while to open up the heart.

Sending a blessing to uplift someone.

Think of the person in your life you've loved the most. I think of my cat when I do this exercise.

1. Empty your mind and take a couple of deep breaths.
2. Focus on the bony part of your chest between the nipples (heart).
3. Breathe in through the heart. Imagine good chi flowing through your heart as you inhale. Bathe the heart in chi.
4. Exhale (breathing out bad chi) through the heart/mind. Picture stagnant chi leaving on exhale.
5. Picture someone you love if they're not there physically.
6. When you get the feeling of love in your heart, send the energy to them with your intention as you let the warmth of a smile spread from your heart. Say 'God bless' inwardly.

'What comes from the heart touches the heart.'

—Shoto Tanemura, Ninpo Grandmaster

APPRECIATION

Count your many blessings. Look around yourself, your life. What do you appreciate?

I have a strong appreciation of the natural world. A beautiful tree, a sunset, wild animals all do it for me. What about your children? Your car? Life? Friends? Even an uplifting TV programme or a song could make you feel gratitude for life. Cultivate appreciation in your life and you'll never have a reason to be sad.

NATURE

Spending time in nature is a good way of replenishing your energy in times of stress.

Getting out in the hills or an ancient forest or after the rain or near the sea are beneficial ways of clearing your personal chi and recharging your internal batteries. Nature has its built-in healing power (chi) and can trigger a shift in mood instantly. Just breathing in the clear air on a mountain top or in an ancient pine forest, for instance, can raise your consciousness to higher and higher levels. Makes you want to look after your environment, doesn't it?

This is why Qi masters in ancient times would retreat to the mountains to meditate and observe the night sky. Fasting on fresh mountain herbs and pure clean spring water they would purge the body of all toxins and malicious thoughts, words and deeds while cultivating the purest chi on the planet. In Japan this practice was referred to as *Misogi*.

VISUALISATION

Relax.

Take a few deep breaths and relax. You may wish to do this exercise after Qi gong practice (*see Fire chapter*).

Picture in your mind a pure clean waterfall in a lush green rainforest in the Amazon.

Spend some time here communing with nature.

This exercise is best done in a quiet setting out of doors but can be done anywhere.

COMPASSIONATE SERVICE

Another way to build up love and respect for your fellow man is to devote some time to a voluntary organisation or charity work.

This could be anything from helping out at church jumble sales to community youth work with troubled teenagers. There is a wide range of organisations out there providing placements in such positions. Help with the aged, under-privileged kids, childcare, disabled people or if you are really stuck (if you are housebound for instance), even caring for a pet can bring a little love and compassion into your life, not to mention companionship.

HEALING

Learning to heal is another great way to build compassion. There are many systems of healing and complementary therapies out there just waiting to be discovered.

To use chi energy to heal look at Qigong, Tai Chi, Yoga, Acupuncture, Reiki, Sekhem, Shiatsu, Spiritual Healing among others. (*See the Useful Addresses section at the end of the book.*)

Void

(Spirit Polishing)

'There can be only one!'
—Highlander

THE VOID: SPIRITUAL OR SUBCONSCIOUS?

As we discussed earlier, the Qi field or Void is the all-encompassing nothingness we call the Universe. So much is not just empty space between people, continents, even the planets. As I said earlier, science is just beginning to grasp what mystics (enlightenment seekers) have said for thousands of years. The universe is not just a mechanical machine but has been proved to be intelligent.

Quantum physics has told us of energy particles and waves reaching out into eternity and Albert Einstein disproved Isaac Newton's theory of the universe. 'All is energy' is the new view starting to come into Western science. This is called the 'holographic' or 'holistic' theory of the universe.

Mystics from all continents and from all times have known that in essence there is only one universe and that we are not separate, in fact we are all component parts of the one. The full realisation of this fact is called Enlightenment.

COLLECTIVE UNCONSCIOUS

Carl Gustav Jung, the psychologist, had many mystic experiences and studied Eastern methods. He called the void the 'collective unconscious' and believed that the thoughts and words of every person who ever lived are recorded there for anyone who wishes to access them.

In the ancient Sanskrit language of India this is called *Akasha* and it is here we go when we pass away from this earthly life. Heaven.

ETERNAL: HISTORICAL

Western society teaches us that we're born, live a few short years and then we die. Worm food!

What's the point? we may ask. A mad scramble for material possessions that we must leave behind one day. The only certainties in life are death and taxes. Or, life's a bitch, then you die!

It hasn't always been this way though. In the past we all went to church for our spiritual well-being. Even though most of us don't now we still find we have a need for spiritual guidance in our lives. During the course of history the human race has always believed in a spiritual universe, a God, but science taught us that this was all nonsense and superstition and so we lost faith and stopped going to church. In all the history of humanity we are probably the only ones who have no faith in anything bigger than ourselves. When you consider that we've only held to this world-view for around the last 400 years, this is a just a speck of dust in the eye of history. This is when science and the church split, science for the physical world and religion for the spirit. At school we learned about duality, everything was separate and if you couldn't prove something by scientific methods then it didn't exist. This caused us to lose even more faith in the church and to abandon our spiritual values.

Also, as the scriptures of all religions will tell you, 'No man is perfect'. Even priests and monks! And so the corruption in religion pushed us farther away. Organised religion became a business like every other business and priests preached their versions of God and the afterlife in vague, hard to grasp terms that were beyond most of us.

Science had become the new God.

Then, at the turn of the last century scientists such as Einstein and Oppenheimer began to work on ever-smaller levels and eventually the old world theory of a separate, mechanical universe started to fall apart with the coming of the new quantum mechanics.

It has taken this long to filter through to the ordinary man in the street, but it seems that both the mystic oneness theory of the universe and the holographic (holistic) view from science are actually one and the same. Science has met spirit!

ASK

To ask the universe for guidance or answers to problems you can use meditation:

1. Have your question ready. Think about what you want to ask and keep it in mind.
2. Relax. Clear your mind by first counting breaths, then watching your breathing.

3. Empty your mind of all thoughts.
4. Listen behind the monkey mind's chatter. Tune into the silence.
5. Ask to be guided or ask for an answer to a question.
6. Wait. Answers or guidance can pop into your head anytime up to 72 hours after asking.

   Be watchful for answers.

COSMIC

The reality of the human body is that it is eternal but also transient. It changes, constantly renewing itself at a cellular level. The body you have now is not the one you were born with. In fact your whole cellular structure renews completely every seven years. Buddhist cosmology states that our bodies are eternal in the sense that once the atoms and molecules that compose our bodies were only cosmic dust. They were once at the heart of a star which exploded, sending debris all across the universe. Some of this dust settled on earth and got into the earth, then into the food chain. The food your parents ate before your conception and during your mother's pregnancy eventually made your body. Know that you are part of this chain—cosmic, eternal and immortal.

Even your thoughts have formed and changed over the years. One aspect of you that stays the same is the spirit, the personality, the spirit, the 'I' inside you. It's only here to learn and evolve.

'We are all made of stars.'

—Moby

WHO WANTS TO LIVE FOREVER?

Mystics from all times and parts of the world (including Jesus) have told us that life is eternal. There is no death. Our spirit is immortal. It is energy and it is part of the one universe or God. In most major religions we are taught the same, but to the naked eye when someone dies they're gone, as we can't see them anymore.

The enlightened person will tell you that in reality the person's life force energy, their spirit, has just passed onto a higher vibration of energy and has discarded their old body as it is no longer needed. They are in fact still around somewhere, as spirit is energy and energy is eternal. We are immortal. In China people who have become enlightened are known as immortals. They live their lives with that consciousness.

Science will also tell you that energy goes on forever.

Enlightenment brings us a certainty that the spirit is eternal and after it there can be no doubt whatsoever.

In recent years hundreds of thousands of studies have been done into reincarnation and near-death experiences. Feel free to read up on this subject, if only to put some of your very human fears of death to rest.

My own experience of this came when I was psychotic. I was seeing things, feeling things and hearing a cacophony of voices. Between me and the outside world was a mad, deranged mind… but my spirit, my life force, my personality was intact!

There is no death, only a change of state.

'A fallen leaf returning to the twig? A butterfly fluttering.'
—Moritake

AWAKENING

At the beginning of the book we did an exercise in our minds to identify the various known parts of our minds. We viewed the Ego, Super-ego and subconscious parts of our minds and I asked, When we picture something in our mind's eye or when we say something to ourselves inwardly, what sees the thing we're picturing, what hears what we think?

Can you see the witness? This is our awareness, the personal aspect of our spirit.

This realisation is a spiritual awakening.

THE WATER CYCLE

A cloud bursts above a mountain and it rains down on the mountain top collecting in puddles and rivulets. They combine to form streams flowing down the mountainside joining other streams and rivers. They flow down into lakes and finally out to sea where they are taken back up to the heavens and become a cloud again.

This is an eternal truth.

THE QUICKENING

On the path to enlightenment you may experience flashes of guidance or strange coincidences and unexpected meaningful events.

In the course of our lives most of us have had funny little 'psychic' happenings. The most common one is when we think of someone and the phone rings and it's them, the person we were thinking about. We are reading a book and just the right piece of information seems to jump out of the page of a book we were just browsing through.

Carl Jung called this 'synchronicity'. In Tibet it is called *Rten Brel* and in Japan, *Kami* (ancestors).

Also when we bump into just the right person at just the right time and the encounter leads to something great. This meaningful coincidence is sometimes called serendipity. Use these coincidences as guidance that you are on the right track. Someone, somewhere is trying to tell you something! Be grateful and see where they lead. I like to think of them as little psychic signposts that tell me I'm 'getting warm'. Use these as an indicator that you are on the right track with your life's mission. It's as if universal forces have gathered and come to your aid.

THE ONE

Oneness, enlightenment, sainthood, *satori*. Just some of the names for universal consciousness. Another approach, a more personal one, is used by psychologists. They refer to 'psychic wholeness' and the way I understand it is as follows.

For me it's about integrating your shadow side—all the horrible little things you deny about yourself and would never want anyone to know. We tend to stuff all these things away in the recesses of our minds, but they don't go away and may surface at a later date and create chaos. When we stuff something away or deny it we create a tension, a contraction in the brain. These tensions build and eventually the mind can rebel against us like a child throwing a tantrum.

Rather than resist and deny and fight, which uses up lots of energy, we can embrace our shadow sides. Stop denying your shadow side and start gradually to accept it, to embrace and make peace with it. Whatever is inside you is a part of you that needs to be integrated so you can become whole. We do this by accepting and surrendering to the universe or that which you may call God. When we embrace the shadow these tensions relax and we clear our minds, generating energy. Remember that nothing really means anything in life other than the meaning we assign to it!

This is not an excuse to go around doing what you like to people—remember that what you send out will come back to you at some point. All is known.

It stands to reason that an ordinary person is more whole than a mentally ill person, right? Then an enlightened person is more whole than an ordinary person too. So if a mentally ill person becomes enlightened then they can become whole again.

This is another 'why' you should try for what I call The One. Normal people aren't whole either, just a little more whole than the mentally ill!

Enlightenment = psychic wholeness = oneness.

A good way to experience a feeling of *satori* or absolute consciousness is to go pebble-hunting on the beach. Cast your eyes on the sand and try to find some beautiful coloured pebbles. You'll find that you become totally absorbed in this search, so much so that for a while nothing exists but your consciousness of your beautiful, natural surroundings. You will have achieved a 'no mind' state. In Japanese martial arts this is known as *Mu*.

> *'Like pebbles on a beach,*
> *Kicked around, displaced by feet.'*
> —Paul Weller

VOID MEDITATION
The six wondrous gateways to enlightenment:
1. Count your breaths: every time you exhale count up 1.
2. Stop counting but follow the breaths in silence. Just watch the rising and falling of your abdomen.
3. Be tranquil. Relax.

4. Watch. Watch your breaths or watch the light play on the back of your eyes.

5. Repeat. If thoughts start to bubble up, repeat steps 1 to 4.

6. Be still. Just be. No thoughts, no mind. Feel the spaciousness, the vastness of the infinite universe above and around your head.

It is said that Buddha attained his enlightenment with this method.

'A heavy snowfall disappears into the sea. What silence!'

—Zen saying

ZHAN ZHUANG 3

Do the standing like a tree postures again (*see pp. 43, 45*) but this time hold each posture for 3 minutes. Quiet the mind, then focus on the vast emptiness of the universe above.

The whole set should take 18 minutes.

#

Now, as we reach the end of our time together I hope I will have inspired you enough to start you out on the road to The One. In future I hope you will refer back to this little book and truly *know* what Enlightenment is about. Rather than a left-brained, intellectual understanding, I hope that your heart will shine with the light of wisdom and compassion as we head through this life to God knows what. These techniques will help you adjust to the new world-view with its speeded-up technology and high stress levels. With determination, one day a beautiful butterfly—your soul—will soar into the void, becoming one with all that is.

You are now a polished gem. Go forward and shine.

I wish you love, health and happiness

'Shine on you crazy diamond.'

—Pink Floyd

Afterword

On 13 September 2001, two days after the 9/11 attacks in the US, I got out of hospital to a changed world. I had been in the Royal Edinburgh for three and a half months under a Section 18.

I was in a daze. I had chronic fatigue and had been told I was suffering from the negative symptoms of schizophrenia. I lay on my back with no energy even to go out for food and essentials. I was sleeping twelve hours a day and all I wanted to do was sit quietly and think things over.

It was around then that my family started to distance themselves from me. I heard every excuse in the book why they couldn't visit and I got tired of it. I think they were scared I'd become dependent on them.

'You could never write a book', they told me, but I put my fingers in my ears and did it anyway. I think half of it was defiance. I used to think of their smug faces if I failed and the anger would spur me on all the more.

This is how I learned the value of self-reliance. The same goes for the illness. You can't leave it all to the doctors and psychiatrists. You have to make an effort to learn about your own condition.

My first novel, *The One*, is based on my actual experiences of schizophrenia and is set mostly in the Royal Edinburgh hospital. It's a psychotic adventure from inside the mind of the sufferer, never before documented in this way. My secret was that I had psychic objectivity, mindfulness. I could 'watch' my thoughts, as I'd learned in cognitive therapy.

There was little else to do in hospital but smoke and watch TV, so I jotted down maps of each episode I went through. I wrote down keywords in little bubbles, describing what happened to me. Then I put them in order and linked them all up, leaving me with a map to work from. I started to write and developed a style as I went along. The funny thing was, I didn't fully understand what *The One* was about when I wrote it. I just wrote what happened to me. It's only in the last few years that I've realised what it was I was being taught. This book hopefully will help you understand the deeper meanings in *The One*. I like to think of us mentally ill people as explorers of the realms of the mind. We should be consulted, not insulted!

As a result of all I've been through, I can honestly say that I'm grateful for all the lessons I've learned. I wouldn't be half the character I am now without the knowledge that hardship has brought me. As a by-product of my suffering, my life force, my spirit, my personality has become stronger and more rounded. I'm now doing a lot of things I never dreamed I could do only a couple of years ago—as a schizophrenic, anxious, paranoid, angry, depressed, deluded, agoraphobic, hypochondriac!

The Way of the Wayward Warrior is a kind of framework, not strict Buddhist or Taoist teachings. It has nothing to do with organised religion. It's a way of living, drawing on global culture and universal consciousness. After a while you learn to become your own teacher, your own psychologist. There is no leader, no middleman, only the Way. No guru, no one to follow. In the end it's between you and He who watches over you.

APPENDIX
Cognitive Behaviour Therapy Sheets

Fill in the blank CBT sheets on the next few pages (or create your own) any time you catch yourself thinking negative thoughts. The sheets will help you home in on any A.N.T.s the monkey mind spits out. Over time you can change your habitual thought process for a more positive outlook.

SITUATION: WHAT I WAS DOING AT THE TIME	SYMPTOMS: HOW I FELT	RATE YOUR SYMPTOMS 1-10	WHAT ARE YOU SAYING TO YOURSELF?	WHAT OTHER WAY COULD YOU SEE THE SITUATION? A MORE POSITIVE, RATIONAL TRUTH...
Example: I was out shopping, the supermarket was very busy.	I started to feel stressed and nervous, I had butterflies in my stomach and my mind was racing.	8 (quite severe)	I need to get out of here. I want to run. I feel faint and if I don't get away from here I'll die.	The symptoms I'm feeling are only anxiety and adrenaline. It can't hurt me so I'll stand my ground no matter how I feel. I can handle this!
I was at home watching TV with my partner. We had an argument.	Angry, in a rage, my blood was boiling, my teeth were clenched.	5 (mid-way)	If I don't get away from here I'll blow. I'm frustrated with trying to explain to her. She won't listen, she's done it to wind me up.	I'm jumping to conclusions and making negative assumptions: these are A.N.T.s. If I indulge in them I'm going to fall out with my partner and I'll feel worse. A.N.T.s are a waste of energy and make me feel ill.
At work, the boss told me off. She says my mind's not on my work.	Down, depressed. I felt helpless, as though I could curl up and die. I wanted to hide away in bed.	6	I'm useless and I always muck everything up. Nobody seems to think I'm good enough. If I lose my job I'll not be able to pay the rent and I'll lose everything. I don't want to live.	I've been in a fog recently. The boss was just having a hard day—she's usually very nice to me. I've been believing A.N.T.s again. Things aren't so bad, I just need to rest and unwind a bit. I'll take a walk along the beach, maybe visit some friends and family—I need to stop living in my head.

SITUATION: WHAT I WAS DOING AT THE TIME	SYMPTOMS: HOW I FELT	RATE YOUR SYMPTOMS 1-10	WHAT ARE YOU SAYING TO YOURSELF?	WHAT OTHER WAY COULD YOU SEE THE SITUATION? A MORE POSITIVE, RATIONAL TRUTH…

SITUATION: WHAT I WAS DOING AT THE TIME	SYMPTOMS: HOW I FELT	RATE YOUR SYMPTOMS 1-10	WHAT ARE YOU SAYING TO YOURSELF?	WHAT OTHER WAY COULD YOU SEE THE SITUATION? A MORE POSITIVE, RATIONAL TRUTH...

FURTHER READING

Geoff Thompson, *Fear, The Friend of Exceptional People* and *The Elephant and the Twig: The Art of Positive Thinking*

Wong Kiew Kit, *The Art of Chi Kung* and *Chi Kung For Health and Vitality*

Anthony Robbins, *Unlimited Power*

Dan Millman, *The Way of the Peaceful Warrior; No Ordinary Moments* and *Everyday Enlightenment*

Shoto Tanemura, *Ninpo Bugei Vol.1: Fundamental Taijutsu*

Miyamoto Musashi, *The Book of Five Rings*

David Servan-Shreiber, *Healing Without Freud or Prozac*

Jesse Lynn Hanley and Nancy Deville, *Tired of Being Tired*

Marius Romme and Sandra Escher, *Accepting Voices*

Diane Stein, *Essential Reiki*

Jack Angelo, *Spiritual Healing*

Thich Nhat Hahn, *Peace Is Every Step*

Elizabeth Kübler Ross, *On Death and Dying*

Stephen K Hayes, *The Mystic Arts of the Ninja*

John Stevens, *The Secrets of Aikido*

H. H. Dalai Lama, *The Art of Happiness*

Michael Talbot, *The Holographic Universe*

USEFUL ADDRESSES

Choose Life is 'a strategy and action plan to reduce suicide in Scotland.'
www.chooselife.net

'The **Scottish Recovery Network** aims to engage communities across Scotland in debate on how best to promote and support recovery from long-term mental health problems.'
www.scottishrecovery.net

'The **Reiki Alliance** is an international community of Reiki Masters.'
www.reikialliance.com

'**Mind** is the leading mental health charity in England and Wales.'
www.mind.org.uk

The **Hearing Voices Network** offers 'information, support and understanding to people who hear voices and those who support them.'
www.hearing-voices.org

The **College of Chi Kung** is 'open to individuals who want to deepen their knowledge of Chi Kung.'
www.collegeofchikung.co.uk

Geoff Thompson is the author of *The Elephant and the Twig* and other self-help books.
www.geoffthompson.com